Ketogenic Diet

21 Days To Rapid Fat Loss, Unstoppable Energy And Upgrade Your Life

Lose Up To a Pound a day

Table of Contents

Introduction

I want to thank you and congratulate you for downloading the book, *"Ketogenic Diet: 21 Day Plan To Rapid Fat Loss, Unstoppable Energy And Upgrade Your Life - Lose Up To a Pound a day"*.

In an attempt to lose weight, many people have tried most if not all diets. The sad part is that most diets don't deliver on their promise and many people gain back all the weight lost once they resume their eating habits. You need to understand that in order to lose weight, you need to overhaul your lifestyle; this means changing the foods you eat, your eating habits and engaging in physical activities.

One diet that seeks to help you do this is the ketogenic diet; this diet emphasizes on eating less carbohydrates (very few), more healthy fats, and adequate protein; hence, helping you lose weight. If you want to learn more about the ketogenic diet, why it works, how it works, how to get started and some mistakes to avoid, this book will help you with all that. It will teach you about the ketogenic diet and answer all questions you may have about the diet.

Thanks again for downloading this book, I hope you enjoy it!

What Is The Ketogenic Diet And Why It Works

The Ketogenic diet is simply a high-fat low-carb diet that offers a number of health benefits including weight loss. For many years, people thought that fat made them fat; hence, this led to many people trying to lose weight by reducing their fat intake by taking low-fat substitutes of different foods. Due to the big wave of 'fat makes you fat', different food manufacturers had to take action to help people 'stop getting fat. They did so by reducing the amount of fat in various foods. There was a problem of food not being tasty as a result of reduced fat levels so these companies had to look for a way of making the low fat food tasty. Here is what they did. To make low-fat food still tasty, they added more sugar. Unfortunately, instead of people losing weight, they actually gained weight. Then you may ask; why is that so?

Well, in the recent past, there have been more studies looking at whether fat actually makes you fat and the conclusion is that sugar is what actually makes you fat. How is that so? When you take a high carb diet, the pancreas releases insulin to make the glucose available to blood cells and to manage blood sugar levels. Insulin facilitates the cells to absorb glucose from the bloodstream, and without it (insulin), the cells would starve of glucose even if the bloodstream has excess of glucose! Generally, the body cells absorb some glucose for use in metabolic activities with the excess glucose being converted to fat for storage. It is important to understand that the body's primary source of fuel is glucose and as long as the body has adequate supply of glucose, it will not burn fat.

The ketogenic diet seeks to put the body in a state where it burns fat for energy (ketosis). When you take a diet low in carb, adequate protein, and high in fat, the level of glucose (the body's primary source of fuel) is low; hence, the body is forced to look for other sources of fuel; hence turning to fats. Thus, ketosis is a metabolic state where fats are broken down in the liver into ketones for energy. We will look at ketosis in much more detail in a later chapter. For now, let us try to understand why the ketogenic diet works and has helped many people lose weight.

Why The Ketogenic Diet Is Effective For Weight Loss

1: According to many people, a few days after withdrawing from carbohydrates, they experienced increased energy levels. Why do you think this is the case? This is because a gram of fat has dense nutritional energy. Once you feel more energetic; then you can engage in different activities including working out to burn fat. In addition, once you start feeling much better, you are unlikely to succumb to emotional eating, which is the main culprit for many people who are overweight and obese.

2: The ketogenic diet also works because it is satiating. As earlier mentioned, a ketogenic diet is high in fat, adequate protein and low in carb. Fats are satiating and so are proteins. Thus, you will feel full for longer and have no need to overeat.

3: The ketogenic diet also works because it helps activate fat metabolism because of drastically reduced level of insulin in the body. Given that you reduce your intake of carbs, your blood has less of glucose, which means that there won't be need for the secretion of high amounts of insulin. Keep in mind that besides facilitating the cells to absorb glucose, insulin has the effect of inhibiting fat metabolism (lipolysis). Instead, it actually promotes fat storage and glycogen accumulation (glycolysis). As such, with reduced insulin levels, your body can effectively start metabolizing fats since there is no inhibition. You can read more here (http://bit.ly/1qcMevw) and here (http://bit.ly/1oBtrZg).

With that understanding of the ketogenic diet, let us now look in depth at what exactly happens to your body when on a ketogenic diet.

What Happens To Your Body While On A Ketogenic Diet?

When you eat a diet high in carbohydrates, your body will break the carbohydrates into glucose to create ATP, which is an energy molecule needed for daily activities. As for the excess glucose, two things happen:

1: Glycogenesis: Any excess glucose is converted to glycogen and stored in muscles and liver. Estimates indicate that half of daily energy is what can be stored as glycogen.

2: Lipogenesis: When your muscles and liver have enough glycogen, the extra will be converted into fat for storage.

When you are on a ketogenic diet, your body will burn fat to create ketones. Ketones are created when your body breaks down fats, which creates fatty acids, which are then burned in the liver in a process referred to as beta-oxidation. The result is creation of ketones, which fuel your brain and muscles. You will be amazed to learn that actually, your brain and body prefer ketones since the body can run 70% more efficiently on ketones than glucose. This is according to a couple of studies.

Let us look at the ketosis process more closely:

When your liver breaks down fat, glycerol and fatty acid molecules are produced. The fatty acids are then broken down further in a process referred to as ketogenesis and a ketone body referred to as acetoacetate is then produced. Acetoacetate is converted into 2 kinds of ketone bodies:

1: Beta-hydroxybutyrate- Acetoacetate is normally converted into this ketone body when you have been on the ketogenic diet for some time. Your brain prefers this ketone.

2: Acetone: This may be metabolized into glucose; although in most cases it is excreted as waste. It usually has a distinct smelly breath.

Over time, the body expels fewer ketone bodies and you may start thinking that ketosis is probably slowing down; this is not the case. The brain is burning the beta-hydroxybutyrate and your body is doing its best to give the brain as much energy as possible. This is why if you are on the ketogenic diet for a while, you will not experience deep levels of ketosis.

How Do You Know You Are In Ketosis? Measuring Ketones

In order to achieve ketosis, you need to have serum ketones between 0.5 and 3.0mM. Below are easy to use home kits that you can use to know your ketone levels.

Blood Ketone Meter
This is the most accurate one to measure Beta-Hydroxybutyrate. Blood ketone meters can determine, with precision, the level of ketones in the blood; however, they are quite expensive. The meter costs around $40 and each test strip costs $5. This means that if you want to measure your ketone levels daily, you will need to part with $150.

Breathalyzer
As mentioned earlier, when on a ketogenic diet, your breath has a distinct smell. A breathalyzer is a cheap way to measure the concentration of acetone. Keep in mind though that breath ketones can vary from blood ketones.

Urine ketone strips
Ketostix and other urine detection strips may not be as effective because they only show the excess ketone bodies being excreted from the body through the urine. However, they are easy to use and affordable.

Observation
You can also listen to your body and determine if you are in ketosis. For instance, when in ketosis, your breath, urine and sweat smell acetone, which is a "fruity" smell. If you detect this, then you are most likely in ketosis.

With that understanding of what happens to your body during ketosis, the question you may want to ask is; how then do you get started on the diet?

Getting Started: Set Yourself Up For Success

In order to get started on the ketogenic diet and be successful at it, you need to do a few things. What are these things?

Set goals

It is important to determine why you want to start on a ketogenic diet. Are you looking to lose weight, build muscle, or maintain lost weight? Determining your 'why' is what will keep you going during those difficult times when you just want to eat something you are not supposed to.

Once you determine why you want to get started on a ketogenic diet, take a second to think why you want to achieve that goal. For instance, if you want to lose weight, why do you want to lose weight? Once you write your reason, go to the computer, search for someone you want to be like physically on Google, print it out, and stick the picture on your mirror so that you see yourself it each time you look in the mirror.

Get an accountability partner

The next thing you want to do is get an accountability partner who will hold you accountable. You can also join different ketogenic forums online for that extra support and encouragement. Also, read as many success stories as possible to be excited that you can actually lose weight.

Restock your pantry

Once you have made your resolve to get started on the ketogenic diet, you have two options as to how you can adopt the diet; you can decide to go cold turkey or start incorporating ketogenic meals into your diet.

If you decide to go cold turkey; then get rid of all processed foods and foods you are not supposed to eat while on a ketogenic diet. The next thing is to restock your pantry with foods that you should eat. We will look at how your grocery list should look like in a subsequent chapter.

If you decide to start incorporating ketogenic meals into your diet, determine what meals you would like to replace with ketogenic meals and how long you want to do this until you fully go ketogenic.

Get ketones measuring kit
It is important to have something that you can use to measure your ketone levels. This will help you know easily when you get into ketosis. It also helps you track your progress while on the ketogenic diet.

Even as you get started on a ketogenic diet, it is important to know about some common mistakes that you are likely to make so that you can avoid them.

Avoid These Mistakes
Avoiding the below mistakes will ensure your success while on the ketogenic diet:

Eating too much protein
Most dieters starting on a low carb diet replace the carbohydrates with protein instead of fat. You need to understand that eating too much protein can lead to gluconeogenesis, which is simply conversion of amino acids to glucose. This is not what you are looking for while on a ketogenic diet; you want to have low glucose levels. The good thing is that once you start increasing your fat intake, your need for protein will reduce.

Not eating enough fat

As mentioned above, many beginners on a ketogenic diet replace what carbohydrates they used to eat with protein rather than fat. Therefore, increase your fat intake. Get fats from omega-rich foods such as fatty fish and foods that have monounsaturated fats like extra virgin olive oil and avocados.

Eating the wrong type of fat

You not only need to increase your fat intake but also eat enough of healthy fats. Thus, stay away from seed and vegetable soils and instead eat saturated fats like coconut oil, butter, and animal fat like tallow as well as monounsaturated fat like olive oil and fish oil.

Eating too many nuts

Nuts provide you with the much-needed fats; however, they are also equally high in calories. 100g of macadamia nuts have over 700 calories. In addition, it is very easy to overeat nuts as opposed to other sources of fat like avocados. What you need to do is to take nuts in moderation. A handful of nuts is all you need to snack on. Also, don't do this daily; you can take nuts thrice a week.

Eating too much of dairy products

While full-fat dairy is high in fat, it is also high in calories and very easy to overeat. In addition, dairy is high in lactose (a type of sugar), which can spike your insulin levels. Opt for dairy products high in fat like cream and butter but low in protein.

Being scared of trying new foods and sticking to the same meals

Starting on a ketogenic diet is a lifestyle change and you are likely to know how to prepare a few meals. This means you may just want to stick to the same old meals and don't want to try something new. Well, the downside with this is that you will be bored within a short time and you are likely to seek what you may consider exciting new meals that are high in carbohydrates. Therefore, make an effort to eat new foods and prepare new recipes weekly or bi-weekly to keep you excited trying new things.

Eating foods labeled "low-carb"

Just eat real food. Avoid buying packaged or prepared foods labeled low-carb because such foods are highly processed and may actually be high in carbohydrates than you think.

Not replenishing sodium

Going on a low-carb diet will definitely reduce your insulin levels. Insulin does a number of other functions other than managing your sugar levels; it also informs the kidneys to hold onto sodium. Since on a low-carb diet, your insulin levels are low, your body starts getting rid of water and sodium. However, sodium is a very important electrolyte in the body and lack of it can lead to fatigue, lightheadedness, constipation, and headaches.

The best way to deal with this is to add more sodium into your body. You can do this by adding salt in your food as well as drinking a cup of broth daily.

Let us now look at how your shopping list should look like.

Grocery List

Include the following foods:

Meat
Beef
Chicken
Pork
Bacon
Salami
Pepperoni
Deli cold cuts
Sausage
Ham
Lamb
Turkey

Fish and Seafood
Salmon
Tuna
Crab
Scallops
Cod
Tilapia
Shrimp

Vegetables
Asparagus
Carrots
Cauliflower
Celery
Bell Pepper
Mushrooms
Green beans

Romaine lettuce
Shallots
Squash
Spinach
Kale
Broccoli
Mushroom
Cabbage
Artichoke hearts
Cucumbers
Arugula
Asparagus

Dairy
Full-fat cheese
Full-fat cream cheese
Butter
Full-fat sour cream
Heavy whipping cream
Greek yogurt

Fruits
Avocado
Strawberries
Blueberries
Cranberries
Blackberries
Raspberries

Nuts and seeds
Walnuts
Pistachios
Macadamias
Hazelnuts
Almonds

Pecans
Flax
Pumpkin
Sunflower
Sesame

Condiments
Lemon juice
Salad dressings
Hot sauce
Mustard
Mayonnaise
Soy sauce

Others
Eggs
Sweeteners like stevia, Splenda erythritol
Herbs
Spices
Nut butters
Unsweetened cocoa powder
Dark chocolate
Unsweetened almond milk
Unsweetened coconut milk

Let us now look at recipes you can prepare with the above ingredients. Before we get to the recipes, we will start with a meal plan that shows you how to follow the ketogenic diet over a period of 4 weeks.

4-Week Ketogenic Meal Plan

In this chapter, we are going to look at a 4-week meal plan that you can adopt to kickstart your ketogenic diet journey.

Week 1

Day 1
Breakfast: 1 cup unsweetened tea with cream and <u>Asparagus frittata</u>
Lunch: <u>Salmon stuffed avocado</u> and 1 cup Greek yogurt
Snack: 1 handful of almonds
Dinner: <u>Bone Broth</u>

Day 2
Breakfast: 1 cup unsweetened coffee with cream and <u>pesto scrambled eggs</u>
Lunch: <u>Shrimp and cauliflower curry</u>
Dinner: <u>Burger with creamed spinach</u>

Day 3
Breakfast: <u>Strawberry almond smoothie</u>
Lunch: Leftovers of previous night's dinner (Burger with creamed spinach)
Dinner: <u>Roasted Pecan Green beans</u>

Day 4
Breakfast: Unsweetened coffee with cream and <u>frittata muffins</u>
Lunch: Leftovers of previous night's dinner (Roasted Pecan Green Beans)
Dinner: <u>Curry rubbed chicken</u> with steamed broccoli

Day 5
Breakfast: Asparagus frittata with 1 cup Greek yogurt

Lunch: Leftovers of previous night's dinner (Curry rubbed chicken with steamed broccoli)
Snack: ½ avocado
Dinner: Beef bone broth

Day 6
Breakfast: Strawberry almond smoothie
Snack: 1 handful walnuts
Lunch: Salmon stuffed avocado with 1 cup Greek yogurt
Dinner: Burger with creamed spinach

Day 7
Breakfast: Pesto scrambled eggs with 1 cup of unsweetened tea
Lunch: Shrimp with cauliflower curry
Dinner: Roasted chicken broth

Week 2

Day 1
Breakfast: Avocado Smoothie
Lunch: Taco tartlets
Dinner: Orange beef stew

Day 2
Breakfast: Keto Breakfast
Lunch: Raspberry avocado smoothie
Snack: 1 boiled egg
Dinner: Salmon with spinach and hollandaise sauce

Day 3
Breakfast: Frittata muffins with 1 cup of unsweetened tea with cream
Lunch: Salmon stuffed avocado
Dinner: Burger with creamed spinach

Day 4
Breakfast: Pesto scrambled eggs
Lunch: Leftovers of burger with creamed spinach
Dinner: Curry rubbed chicken with steamed vegetables

Day 5
Breakfast: Keto breakfast
Lunch: Raspberry avocado smoothie
Snack: 1 handful pumpkin seeds
Dinner: Orange beef stew

Day 6
Breakfast: Bacon burger
Lunch: Taco tartlets
Dinner: Curry rubbed chicken with steamed broccoli

Day 7

Breakfast: Frittata muffins with 1 cup green tea
Lunch: Leftovers of previous night's dinner (curry rubbed chicken with steamed broccoli)
Dinner: Burger with creamed spinach

Week 3

Day 1
Breakfast: Scrambled eggs
Lunch: Avocado olive Salad
Dinner: Slow cooker chicken broth

Day 2
Breakfast: Asparagus frittata
Lunch: Shrimp and cauliflower curry
Dinner: Roasted pecan green beans

Day 3
Breakfast: Avocado smoothie
Snack: 1 handful mixed berries
Lunch: Leftovers of previous night's dinner (roasted pecan green beans)
Dinner: Orange beef stew

Day 4
Breakfast: Keto breakfast
Lunch: Taco tartlets
Dinner: Burger with creamed spinach

Day 5
Breakfast: Scrambled eggs
Lunch: Shrimp and cauliflower curry
Dinner: Salmon with spinach and hollandaise sauce

Day 6
Breakfast: Blackberry smoothie
Lunch: Avocado olive salad
Dinner: Pork chop bone broth

Day 7
Breakfast: Asparagus frittata

Lunch: <u>Raspberry avocado smoothie</u>
Snack: ½ avocado
Dinner: <u>Curry rubbed chicken with steamed vegetables</u>

Week 4

Day 1
Breakfast: <u>Scrambled eggs</u> with 1 cup green tea
Lunch: <u>Chocolate raspberry smoothie</u>
Snack: 1 handful berries
Dinner: <u>Burger with creamed spinach</u>

Day 2
Breakfast: <u>Pesto scrambled eggs</u>
Lunch: <u>Avocado tuna bites</u>
Dinner: <u>Spinach salad</u>

Day 3
Breakfast: <u>Ketogenic chocolate smoothie</u>
Lunch: <u>Baked salmon</u> with vegetables
Dinner: Burger with creamed spinach

Day 4
Breakfast: <u>Asparagus Frittata</u>
Lunch: Leftovers of previous night's dinner (burger with creamed spinach)
Dinner: <u>Lemon chicken broth</u>

Day 5
Breakfast: <u>Blueberry smoothie</u>
Snack: ½ avocado
Lunch: <u>Baked salmon</u>
Dinner: Spinach salad

Day 6
Breakfast: <u>Bacon burger</u>
Lunch: <u>Shrimp in garlic sauce</u>
Dinner: <u>Curry rubbed chicken</u> with steamed vegetables

Day 7

Breakfast: Keto breakfast
Lunch: Leftovers of previous night's dinner (curry rubbed chicken with steamed vegetables)
Dinner: Dark chicken broth

Breakfast

1. Keto Breakfast

Serves 1

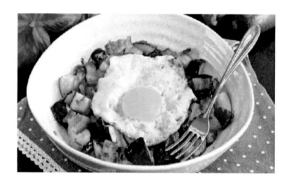

Ingredients
1 tablespoon butter
½ avocado
2 large portobello mushrooms
5 thin bacon slices
1 egg
Salt to taste
Freshly ground black pepper

Directions
1. Heat half the butter in a pan over medium heat.
2. Add mushrooms, sprinkle salt and pepper and cook for around 8 minutes or until cooked.
3. Fry the bacon and egg in a separate pan since the mushroom will release moisture.
4. Once ready, serve and enjoy.

Nutritional Information per serving
489 calories, 41.3 g fats, 6.6 g net carbs, and 19.5 g protein

2. Asparagus Frittata

Serves 4

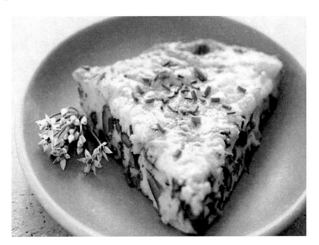

Ingredients

20 small asparagus spears

10 eggs

5 oz. soft goat cheese

¼ cup full-fat heavy whipping cream

1 large red bell pepper

1 small shallot

2 small spring onions

Freshly ground black pepper

Salt to taste

2 tablespoons ghee

1 tablespoon fresh tarragon

2 tablespoons fresh mint

2 tablespoons fresh parsley

3.5 oz. bacon

4 cherry tomatoes to serve

Directions

1. Preheat oven to 400 degrees F.

2. Cut the asparagus stem off.

3. Wash, deseed, and slice the bell pepper into small strips. Peel and chop the spring onion and shallot finely.

4. Use a tablespoon of ghee to grease a non-stick pan and then add the vegetables you prepared in the previous step. Season with salt.

5. Cook for 5 minutes then whisk the eggs, herbs and cream in a bowl.

6. Transfer the cooked vegetables in a baking dish, pour the egg mixture on top, and sprinkle with the cheese.

7. Place in the oven and cook for around 20 minutes.

8. Remove the dish from the oven, put the bacon on the frittata, return to the oven and cook for an additional 20 minutes.

9. In the mean time, prepare the tomatoes. Grease a pan over medium heat with a tablespoon of ghee. Add the tomatoes to the pan and roast for 5 minutes.

10. Serve the frittata with the tomatoes and enjoy.

Nutritional Information per serving

503 calories, 37.5 g fats, 6.3g net carbs, and 25.5g protein

3. Frittata Muffins

Serves 8

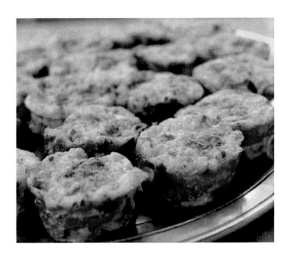

Ingredients
¼ teaspoon salt
½ teaspoon pepper
2 teaspoons dried parsley
1 tablespoon butter
½ cup cheddar cheese
4 oz. bacon
½ cup half and half
8 large eggs

Directions

1. Preheat the oven to 375 degrees.

2. Mix half and half and eggs in a bowl.

3. Fold in the cheese, bacon and spices and add the rest of the ingredients.

4. Use butter to grease a muffin tin.

5. Pour the mixture into each cup making sure you fill ¾ way.

6. Put in the oven and cook for 15 minutes or until golden brown on the edges.

7. Remove from the oven and cool before serving.

Nutritional Information per serving

205 calories, 16.1g fats, 1.3g net carbs, and 13.6g protein

4. Scrambled Eggs

Serves 1

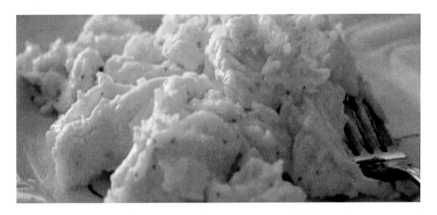

Ingredients
1 oz. cheddar cheese
2 tablespoons butter
2 large eggs, beaten

Directions
1. Heat a pan over medium heat, and add butter.
2. When the butter has melted, add the eggs. Let the eggs cook only turning them once or twice.
3. Add cheese and mix.

Nutritional Information per serving
453 calories, 43g fats, 1.2g net carbs, and 19g protein

5. Bacon Burger

Serves 1

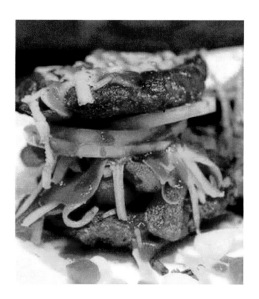

Ingredients
2 tablespoons cheddar cheese

¼ teaspoon Worcestershire

¼ teaspoon onion powder

½ teaspoon salt

¾ teaspoon soy sauce

½ teaspoon black pepper

½ teaspoon minced garlic

1 ½ teaspoons chopped chives

2 slices bacon

200g ground beef

Directions

1. Cook the bacon in a skillet until crisp.

2. Once ready, remove from skillet, put on a paper towel, drain the grease and put aside.

3. Combine bacon, beef and spices in a large bowl.

4. Form three patties then put 2 tablespoons of the bacon fat on the skillet.

5. Once the fat is hot, put the patties and cook each side for 4 minutes or depending on how you want it.

6. Remove the patties from the skillet and allow to rest for 3 minutes.

7. Assemble the burger starting with one patty, then bacon and some cheese, another patty, bacon and cheese and the final patty on top. Sprinkle cheese on top.

Nutritional Information per serving

649 calories, 51.8g fats, 1.8g net carbs, and 43.5g Protein

6. Pesto Scrambled eggs

Serves 1

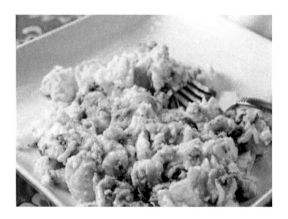

Ingredients
3 organic eggs
Freshly ground black pepper
Salt to taste
2 tablespoons sour cream
1 tablespoon pesto
1 tablespoon butter

Directions
1. Beat eggs in a bowl; season with pepper and salt.
2. Heat a pan over medium heat, add butter; once hot, pour the eggs into the pan.
3. Cook on low heat and stir constantly. Add the pesto and mix.
4. Remove from heat, add cream, and mix with eggs. This will make the eggs have a creamy mixture.

Nutritional Information per serving
467 calories, 41.5 g fats, 2.6 g net carbs, and 20.4 g protein

Lunch Recipes

7. Shrimp and Cauliflower Curry

Serves 6

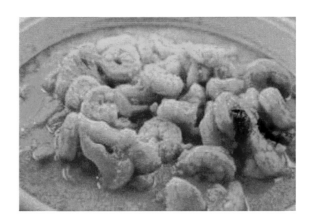

Ingredients
½ head cauliflower
24oz. shrimp
¼ teaspoon Xanthan gam
2 tablespoons curry powder
3 tablespoons olive oil
¼ cup heavy cream
¼ cup butter
1 cup coconut milk
1 medium onion
4 cups chicken stock
¼ teaspoon cinnamon
¼ teaspoon cardamom
½ teaspoon turmeric
½ teaspoon coriander
½ teaspoon ground ginger
1 teaspoon paprika
1 teaspoon cayenne pepper
1 teaspoon onion powder

1 teaspoon chili powder

2 teaspoons garlic powder

1 tablespoon cumin

1 tablespoon coconut flour

5 cups raw spinach

Directions

1. Mix the spices and put aside.

2. Cut the onion then put into a pan with 3 tablespoons olive oil. Heat over medium heat and cook the onion until translucent.

3. Add spices, xanthan, cream and butter and stir until well mixed.

4. After about 2 minutes of cooking add coconut milk and stock; stir, cover and cook for 30 minutes on low heat.

5. Cut the cauliflower into florets and add to curry. Cook for 15 more minutes while covered.

6. Devein the shrimp and add to curry; cook for 20 minutes while uncovered.

7. Add xanthan gum and coconut flour into the curry and stir. Cook for five more minutes, add spinach, cook for an additional fives minutes and serve.

Nutritional Information per serving

331 calories, 19.5g fats, 5.6g net carbs, 27.4g protein

8. Taco Tartlets

Yields 11 tartlets

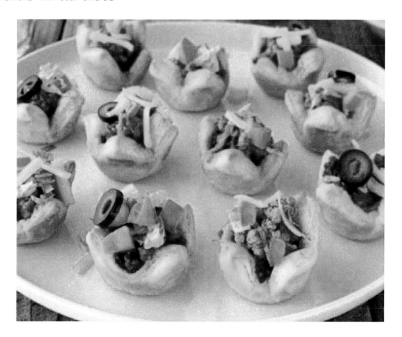

Ingredients

The pastry
3 tablespoons coconut flour
2 tablespoons ice water
¼ teaspoon cayenne
¼ teaspoon paprika
1 teaspoon oregano
¼ teaspoon salt
5 tablespoons butter
1 cup blanched almond flour
1 teaspoon Xanthan gum

Filling
½ teaspoon pepper
1/3 cup cheese
1 teaspoon cumin
2 teaspoons garlic
2 teaspoons yellow mustard
1 tablespoon olive oil
2 tablespoons tomato paste
3 stalks spring onion
80g mushroom
400g ground beef
¼ teaspoon cinnamon
1 teaspoon Worcestershire
1 teaspoon salt

Directions
1. Combine all the pastry dry ingredients in a food processor.
2. Add in butter and pulse until crumbly. Ad the ice water and pulse once more.
3. Put the dough in the freezer for 10 minutes. Remove from the freezer and use a rolling pin to roll out.
4. Use a cookie cutter to cut circles. Put the dough in a whoopee pan and preheat the oven to 325 degrees F.
5. Prepare the filling ingredients; slice mushrooms, chop onions and mince garlic.
6. Sauté the onions in olive oil. Add garlic and cook once more.
7. Add ground beef, dry spices, mushrooms and Worcestershire and mix.
8. Add mustard and tomato paste just before you finish.
9. Spoon the beef mixture into the pastry, sprinkle cheese, and bake for 30 minutes.

Nutritional Information per tartlet
241 calories, 19.4g fats, 1.7g net carbs, and 13.1g protein

9. Salmon Stuffed Avocado

Serves 2

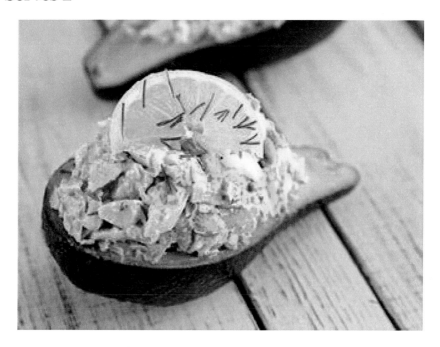

Ingredients
1 large avocado
1-2 tablespoons chopped dill
1 tablespoon ghee
Freshly ground black pepper
2 salmon fillets
2 tablespoons lemon juice
¼ cup sour cream
1 finely chopped white onion
Lemon wedges to garnish
¼ teaspoon salt

Directions

1. Preheat oven to 400 degrees F. Line a baking tray with parchment paper and put the salmon on top; drizzle with melted ghee. Season with pepper and salt and drizzle with lemon juice. Cook in the oven for 20 minutes

2. Once ready, remove from oven and allow to cool for around 5 minutes. Shred the salmon using a fork and discard the skin.

3. Mix the salmon with sour cream, dill and onion. Squeeze some lemon juice on top and season with pepper and salt.

4. Cut the avocado into half and scoop a little of the avocado flesh into the bowl with salmon and mix.

5. Spoon the above mixture into each avocado half and garnish with lemon wedges.

Nutritional Information per serving

463 calories, 34.6 g fats, 6.4 g net carbs, and 27 g protein

10. Avocado Olive Salad

Serves 2

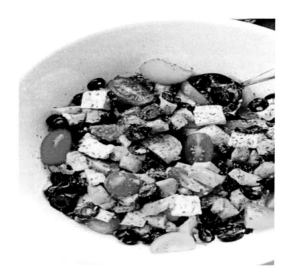

Ingredients
6 olives
1 avocado
2 tablespoons extra virgin olive oil
2 tablespoons pesto
125g mozzarella for salads
3 medium tomatoes

Directions
1. Wash and cut the tomatoes.
2. Cut the avocado in half, deseed and sliced.
3. Halve the olives. Put the tomatoes, avocado and olives into a bowl.
4. Add the olive oil, pesto and mozzarella; season with pepper and salt and enjoy

Nutritional information per serving
581 calories, 50.7 g fats, 8.6 g net carbs, 19.2 g protein

Avocado Tuna Bites
Yields 12 Bites

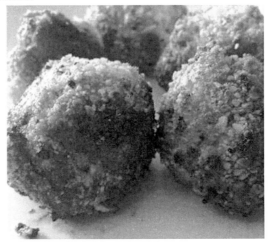

Ingredients
10oz. drained canned tuna
½ cup coconut oil for frying
1/3 cup almond flour
1.4 cup parmesan cheese
1 cubed avocado
¼ cup mayonnaise
Salt and pepper to taste
¼ teaspoon onion powder
½ teaspoon garlic powder

Directions
1. Add tuna and all ingredients except coconut oil and avocado into a bowl and mix.
2. Add the avocado into the bowl and fold into the tuna.
3. Form balls and roll in almond flour.
4. Over medium heat, heat a pan. Add coconut oil and once the oil is hot, fry the balls until browned.
5. Serve and enjoy.

Nutritional Information per tuna bite
135 calories, 11.g fat, 0.8g net carbs, 6.2g protein

11. Shrimp in garlic sauce

Serves 2

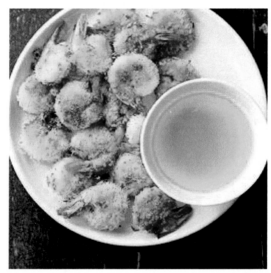

Ingredients
½ lb. shrimp, peeled and deveined
Salt and pepper to taste
½ teaspoon cayenne
3 garlic cloves
¼ cup olive oil
1 lemon wedge

Directions
1. Pour olive oil in a small pan. Add garlic and cayenne.
2. Cook the garlic until fragrant.
3. Cook the shrimp for 2 minutes on each side, season with pepper and salt and squeeze some lemon juice onto the shrimp.
4. Serve the shrimp with the garlic sauce.

Nutritional Information per serving
335 calories, 2.5g net carbs, 27g fat, 22.3g protein

12. Baked Salmon

Serves 4

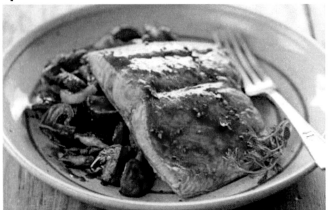

Ingredients
2lbs. salmon fillets
½ cup chopped green onions
½ cup chopped mushrooms
4oz. butter
¼ teaspoon tarragon
½ teaspoon rosemary
¼ teaspoon thyme
1 teaspoon oregano leaves
½ teaspoon basil
½ teaspoon ground ginger
1 teaspoon minced garlic
½ cup tamari soy sauce
4oz. sesame oil

Directions

1. Cut the salmon into ½ lb pieces.

2. Stir together spices, sesame oil and tamari sauce in a bowl. Put the salmon in a Ziploc bag and pour the sauce on top of the salmon.

3. Refrigerate in the marinade for at least 1 hour.

4. Preheat the oven to 350 degrees Fahrenheit. Use foil to line a baking pan.

5. Pour the fillets into the baking pan, arranging the fish in a single layer. Bake the salmon for 10 minutes.

6. As the salmon cooks, prepare the vegetables.

7. Melt butter, add vegetables, and mix to coat in butter.

8. Remove salmon from oven, pour butter mixture over salmon, and bake for about 10 minutes. Once ready, serve immediately.

Nutritional Information per serving

353 calories, 1g net carb, 23g fat, 32g protein

Dinner Recipes

13. Salmon with Spinach and Hollandaise Sauce

Serves 1

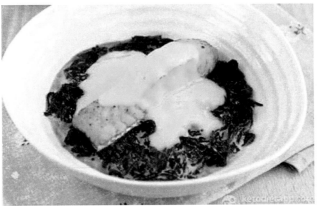

Ingredients
1 salmon fillet
1 serving hollandaise sauce
4.4oz. fresh spinach
Freshly ground black pepper
2 tablespoons ghee
Salt to taste
1 tablespoon heavy whipping cream

Directions

1. Preheat the oven to 400 degrees F and put the salmon on a baking tray. Drizzle half the ghee; season with pepper and salt and cook in the oven for 20 minutes.

2. In the meantime, prepare the spinach. Wash spinach and pat dry the spinach with a paper towel to remove any excess water.

3. Grease a pan with ghee and heat over medium heat. Add the spinach and cook for around 3 minutes; season with salt.

4. Add the whipping cream to the spinach, stir and remove from heat; set aside.

5. Put the salmon on a plate, top with spinach and hollandaise sauce.

Nutritional Information per serving

813 calories, 72.6 g fats, 3.7 g net carbs, and 34 g protein

14. Spinach Salad

Serves 1

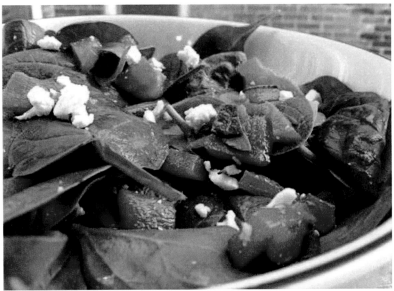

Ingredients
3 cups spinach
1 ½ tablespoons parmesan cheese
½ teaspoon red pepper flakes
2 tablespoons Ranch dressing

Directions
1. Add spinach into a mixing bowl and add the dressing.
2. Mix everything then add red pepper flakes and parmesan.
3. Mix again and serve immediately.

Nutritional Information per serving
208 calories, 18g fats, 3.5g net carbs, and 8g protein

15. Orange Beef Stew

Serves 1 (with leftovers)

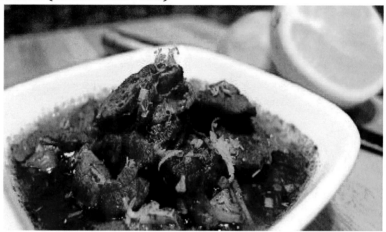

Ingredients
1/4lb beef
Juice of ¼ orange
¼ medium onion
1 tablespoon coconut oil
¾ cup beef broth
1 bay leaf
¼ teaspoon sage
¼ teaspoon rosemary
½ teaspoon fish sauce
½ teaspoon soy sauce
½ teaspoon ground cinnamon
¾ teaspoon minced garlic
¾ teaspoon thyme
Zest of ¼ orange

Directions

1. Cut the meat and vegetables into 1-inch cubes. Season the meat with pepper and salt.

2. Heat coconut oil in a skillet over medium heat. Once hot, add the meat into the skillet; do this in batches, don't overfill.

3. Brown the meat for 2 minutes.

4. Once you have finished browning the meat, add orange juice to deglazed then add the other ingredients except the thyme, sage and rosemary.

5. Let this cook for a few minutes, then transfer all ingredients to a crockpot.

6. Cook on high or 3 hours.

7. Open the crockpot, add the spices and cook for 1 hour.

8. Serve when hot.

Nutritional Information per serving

649 calories, 44.5g fats, 1.9g net carbs, and 53.5g protein

16. Curry Rubbed Chicken

Serves 1

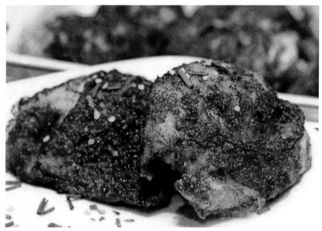

Ingredients
2 chicken thighs
1 pinch ginger
1 pinch cinnamon
1 pinch cardamom
1/8 teaspoon coriander
1/8 teaspoon chili powder
1/8 teaspoon allspice
1/8 teaspoon cayenne pepper
¼ teaspoon garlic powder
¼ teaspoon paprika
¼ teaspoon cumin
½ teaspoon salt
½ teaspoon yellow curry
1 tablespoon olive oil

Directions
1. Preheat oven to 425 degrees F.
2. Mix spices in a bowl, then line a baking sheet with foil and lay the chicken on the foil.
3. Rub the olive oil on the chicken then rub the spice mixture, making sure you coat the chicken liberally.
4. Bake for 4 minutes. Allow it to cool or 5 minutes before you serve.

Nutritional Information per serving
555 calories, 39.8g fats, 1.3g net carbs, and 42.3g protein

17. Roasted Pecan Green Beans

Serves 3 (with leftovers)

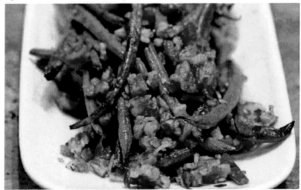

Ingredients
¼ cup chopped pecans
½ lb. green beans
Zest of ½ lemon
½ teaspoon red pepper flakes
1 teaspoon minced garlic
2 tablespoons parmesan cheese
2 tablespoons olive oil

Directions
1. Preheat oven to 450 degrees F.
2. Process the pecans in a food processor until they are chopped nicely.
3. Mix green beans, red pepper flakes, garlic, parmesan cheese, olive oil, zest and pecans in a large bowl.
4. Spread out the mixture onto a baking sheet lined with foil and bake in the oven for 20-25 minutes.
5. Allow to cool for a few minutes before serving.

Nutritional Information per serving
182 calories, 16.8g fats, 3.3g net carbs, and 3.7g protein

Burger with creamed spinach
Serves 2

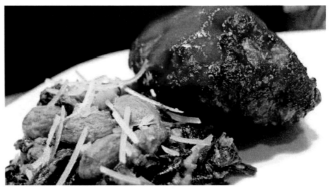

Ingredients
2 ½ cups raw spinach
1lb. ground beef
1 teaspoon cumin
½ tablespoon chipotle seasoning
½ tablespoon butter
½ tablespoon heavy cream
1 tablespoon cream cheese
2 ½ tablespoons roasted almonds
1 teaspoon red pepper flakes
¼ bell pepper
¼ onion
1 cup sliced mushrooms

Directions

1. Preheat oven to 450 degrees F.
2. Put the bell pepper, onion and mushrooms in a food processor and pulse until the vegetables are diced.
3. Add the vegetables, meat (put aside a small amount of meat) and seasonings to a bowl and mix.
4. Form 3 burger patties and place the patties on rack over a baking sheet that has been lined with foil to catch drippings and cook in the oven or 20 minutes.
5. In the meantime, add the remaining meat to a pan and once it begins to sizzle add spinach and red pepper flakes; season with salt and pepper.
6. Once the spinach has wilted add butter, cream cheese almonds and heavy cream and stir. Allow this to cook down and keep warm.
7. Once the burgers are ready, remove from the oven and serve with the spinach.

Nutritional Information per serving

562 calories, 38.5g fats, 4.8g net carbs, and 45.3g protein

Keto Smoothies

18. Avocado Smoothie

Serves 2

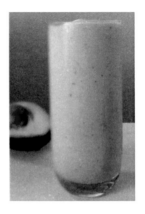

Ingredients
1 ripe avocado
1-2 tablespoons of sweetener
½ cup ice cubes
A few drops vanilla extract
30ml heavy cream
2 cups unsweetened almond milk

Directions
1. Cut avocado in half and deseed. Scoop the avocado flesh into the blender.
2. Add the other ingredients into the blender and blend until creamy and smooth.
3. Serve and enjoy.

Nutritional Information per serving:
243 calories, 4g net carbs, 23g fat, 4g protein

19. Strawberry Almond Smoothie

Serves 2

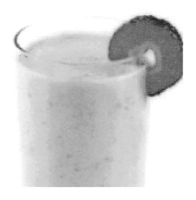

Ingredients
1 scoop whey vanilla powder
¼ cup frozen unsweetened strawberries
4 ounces heavy cream
1 packet stevia
16 ounces unsweetened almond milk

Directions
Put all ingredients in the blender and blend until smooth and creamy. If it is too thick, you can add a little water

Nutritional Information per serving:
304 calories, 6g net carbs, 25g fat, 15g protein

20. Raspberry Avocado Smoothie

Serves 2

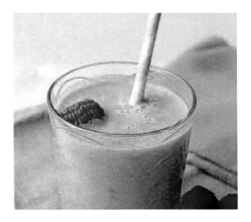

Ingredients
½ cup frozen unsweetened raspberries
1 packet stevia
3 tablespoons lemon juice
1 1/3 cup water
1 ripe peeled avocado, pit removed

Directions
1. Add the ingredients into a blender and blend until smooth.
2. Pour into two glasses and enjoy.

Nutritional Information per serving
227 calories, 4g net carbs, 20g fat, 2.5g protein

21. Blackberry Smoothie

Serves 1

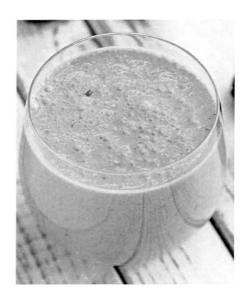

Ingredients
½ cup frozen or fresh black berries
1 teaspoon vanilla extract
1 tablespoon extra virgin coconut oil
½ cup water
¼ cup coconut milk
¼ cup full-fat cream cheese
3-5 drops liquid stevia (optional)

Directions
1. Add all ingredients into a blender.
2. Pulse until smooth. Pour into a glass and enjoy.

Nutritional Information per serving
515 calories, 6.7g net carbs, 53g fat, 6.4g protein

22. Chocolate Raspberry Smoothie

Serves 2

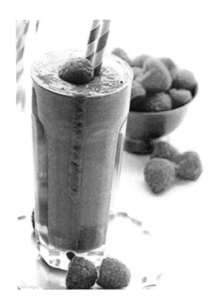

Ingredients
1 tablespoon cocoa powder
1/3 cup frozen raspberries
½ avocado
1 ¼ cups cashew milk
1/8 teaspoon raspberry extract
1 tablespoon powdered swerve sweetener

Directions
1. Put all ingredients in blender and blend until smooth. If you want a thinner consistency, you can add more cashew milk.

Nutritional Information per serving
133 calories, 4.84g net carbs, 9.5g fat, 5.81g protein

23. Ketogenic Chocolate Smoothie

Serves 1

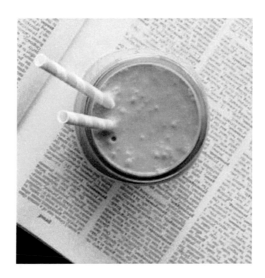

Ingredients
2 free range eggs or 2 tablespoons chia seeds
¼ cup water
½ cup ice
3-5 drops stevia extract
1 tablespoon unsweetened cacao powder
1 tablespoon extra virgin coconut oil
¼ cup whey protein
1 cup heavy whipping cream
½ teaspoon cinnamon

Directions
1. Put all ingredients in the blender beginning with the eggs.
2. Pulse until the mixture is smooth.
3. Serve immediately.

Nutritional Information per serving
570 calories, 4.4g net carbs, 46g, 3.5g protein

24. Blueberry Smoothie

Serves 1

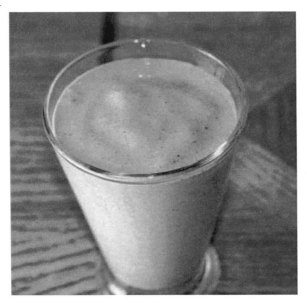

Ingredients
¼ cup frozen blueberries
1 scoop vanilla protein powder
1 cup loosely packed spinach
1/3 cup unsweetened almond milk
½ cup Greek yogurt
1/3 cup ice

Directions
1. Add all ingredients except ice and blend. Add the ice and blend once more.
2. Serve cold.

Nutritional Information per serving
290 calories, 9g net carbs 13.5g fat, 11g protein

Bone Broth Recipes

25. Bone Broth

Makes 6-8 cups

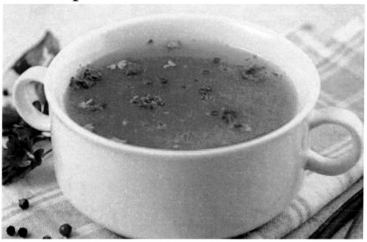

Ingredients

3.3lb oxtail mixed with assorted bones
8-10 cups water or enough to cover bones (do not exceed 2/3
capacity of the pressure cooker, ¾ capacity of slow cooker and
Dutch oven
1 tablespoon salt
2-3 bay leaves
2 tablespoons fresh lemon juice
5 peeled cloves garlic
1 white onion with skin on
2 medium celery stalks
1 medium parsnip
2 medium carrots

Directions

1. Peel the root vegetables and cut then halve the garlic cloves and onion (keep skin on).
2. Cut celery into thirds, put the vegetables into pressure cooker, and add the bay leaves.
3. Add the oxtail and the bones.
4. Add water, lemon juice, and salt.
5. Lock lid and heat over high heat to reach high pressure. Once it reaches high pressure, reduce the heat and set the timer for 90 minutes.
6. Once ready, remove from heat and allow the pressure to release naturally for around 10-15 minutes.
7. Remove the lid and the large bits and pour the broth into a large dish through a strainer. Discard the vegetables.
8. You can drink the broth immediately or freeze.

Nutritional Information per cup:
72 calories, 0.7g net carbs, 6g fat, 3.6g protein

26. Beef Bone Broth

Serves 4

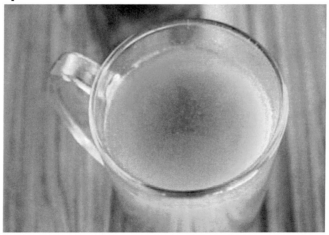

Ingredients
1 bunch flat parsley, chopped
1 teaspoon dried and crushed peppercorns
1 sprig fresh thyme
3 celery ribs
3 coarsely chopped carrots
3 coarsely chopped onions
½ cup cider vinegar
4 quarts water
3 lbs. rib
4 lbs. beef marrow (and knuckle bones)

Directions

1. Put the bones in a large pot. Add vinegar and cover with water. Allow this to stand for 1 hour.

2. In the meantime, put the meaty bones in a roasting pan. Heat the oven to 350 degrees F, and brown the meat in the oven.

3. Once browned, add to the large pot as well as the vegetables. Pour any fat from the roasting pan into the pot. Add water to the roasting pan and stir with wooden spoon to get rid of the browned bits. Add this liquid to the pot.

4. Add more water just to cover the bones. Bring the pot to a boil.

5. Remove any frothy scum that arises to the top. Lower the heat and add crushed peppercorns and thyme.

6. Simmer for at least 2 hours. Just before you finish simmering, add parsley and then simmer for another 10 minutes.

7. Use a slotted spoon to remove bones, and then strain the stock through a mesh strainer into a bowl.

8. Enjoy the broth or let the broth cool, remove fat at the top, transfer to small containers and freeze until when you want to use.

Nutritional information per serving
780 calories, 9g net carbs, 48g fat, 70g protein

27. Roasted Chicken Broth

Serves 4

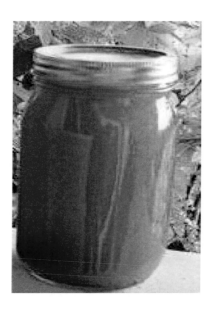

Ingredients
1lb chicken, giblets removed
2 quarts cold water
1 tablespoon ketchup
3 cloves garlic, lightly smashed
2 teaspoons kosher salt
1 rib celery, cut in chunks
1 onion, peeled and quartered

Directions

1. Preheat oven to 400 degrees F.

2. Put celery, onion, and chicken in the Dutch oven and sprinkle salt on top of the chicken.

3. Roast the chicken while uncovered in the oven until the chicken is not pink inside and the skin has browned. This should take around 45 minutes to an hour.

4. Transfer the chicken to the plate until it is cool enough to handle. Once it is cool enough, pick meat from bones and set aside the meat in bowl for other uses.

5. Remove chicken fat from the Dutch oven and leave the browned bits at the bottom.

6. Put the Dutch oven over medium heat, return chicken bones and dark meat from thighs and drumsticks to the pot. Add ketchup, cloves and water and bring to a boil.

7. Scrap the bottom bits using a spoon to dissolve the flavor bits, then reduce the heat and simmer for around 3 minutes, adding water when necessary to maintain the same level.

8. As the broth simmers, skim off and discard any foam that arises to the surface.

9. Once ready, remove, discard meat, vegetables and bones and strain the broth through a sieve and serve or use in other recipes.

Nutritional Information per serving:

421 calories, 7.5gnet carbs, 25.8g fat, 37.6g Protein

28. Slow Cooker Chicken Broth

Serves 5

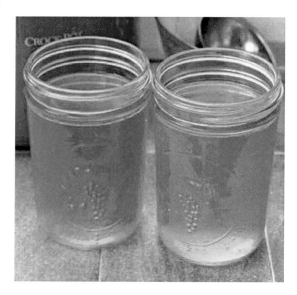

Ingredients
2 chopped carrots
2 ½ lbs bone-in chicken
1 tablespoon dried basil
1 quartered onion
2 celery stalks, chopped
6 cups water

Directions
1. Place the onion, chicken celery, carrots, basil and water in a slow cooker.
2. Cook at low heat for 8-10 hours, discard the vegetables, meat, and strain.
3. Serve and drink or store for later use.

Nutritional Information per serving:
274 calories, 5.8g net carbs, 14.8g fat, 21.7g Protein

29. Pork Chop Broth

Serves 2

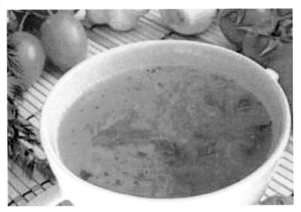

Ingredients
1 clove garlic
1 bone-in pork chop
¼ onion
4 cups water
2 teaspoons chicken base

Directions
1. Cut fat and bones from pork chop and cut the meat into small chunks.
2. Put the fat, meat, and bones in a pan; add chicken base, onion, garlic and water and bring to a boil.
3. Reduce the heat and simmer on low for about 5-6 hours ensuring that you add water every hour.
4. Strain the broth into a bowl and separate bones from meat. Put the meat and ½ of the broth into your blender and blend.
5. Return broth to saucepan and mix well. Serve.

Nutritional Information per serving:
120 calories, 2.7g net carbs, 5g Fat, 15g Protein

30. Lemon Chicken Broth

Serves 6

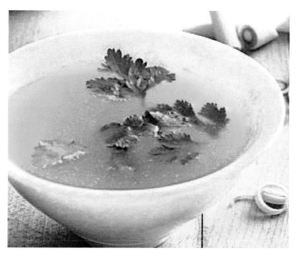

Ingredients
2lbs bone-in, skin on chicken leg quarters
¼ cup fresh cilantro leaves
½ teaspoon salt
1 teaspoon black peppercorns
1 tablespoon chopped garlic
4 (¼ -inch) slices fresh ginger, peeled
3 stalks lemongrass
8 cups water

Directions

1. Put the chicken and water in a Dutch oven and boil. Make sure you skim and discard any foam.

2. Once it boils, lower the heat.

3. Trim the root end of the lemongrass stacks and get rid of the outer tougher leaves. Smash the stalks using the flat side of a knife.

4. Add the peppercorns, garlic, ginger and lemon grass to the pan. Cover partially and simmer for 50 minutes; ensure you skim and discard foam as needed.

5. Using a slotted spoon, remove the chicken from the pan and reserve for later use.

6. Strain the broth and discard the solids. Cool, cover and chill overnight or at least for 8 hours. Skim the fat on the surface and discard.

7. Heat broth in a pan, stir in salt and the sprinkle the cilantro leaves, and serve.

Nutritional information per serving:

19 calories, 0.3g net carbs, 0.6g fat, 3.1g protein

31. Dark Chicken Broth

Yields 2 quarts

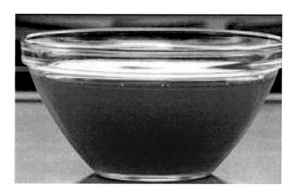

Ingredients
3 roughly chopped celery stalks
2lbs. chicken wings or chicken bones
1 tablespoon olive oil
3 peeled and chopped carrots
1 chopped onion

Directions
1. Preheat the oven to 350 degrees F, then put the vegetables and bones in a roasting pan and toss with the oil. Roast these until browned; it should take around 30 minutes.
2. Transfer the vegetables and bones to a large pot and add 4 quarts water. Bring this mixture to a boil and make sure to skim off any foam forming at the top.
3. Once it boils, reduce the heat and simmer for about 3 hours.
4. Strain the mixture and take the broth or let it cool and freeze for later use.

Nutritional Information per serving:
41 calories, 1.3g net carbs, 1.5g fat, 5.6g protein

Conclusion

Thank you again for downloading this book!

I hope this book has taught you more about the ketogenic diet, how to adopt the diet and be successful. What you need to do next is to determine why you want to get started on the ketogenic diet. Once you do this, you can then restock your pantry and adopt the 4-week meal plan.

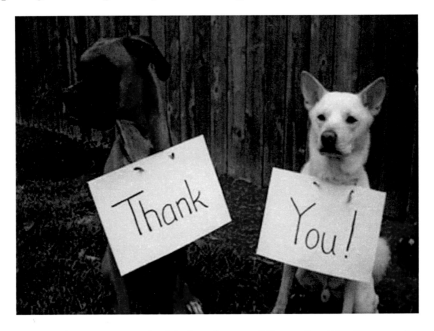

Finally, if you enjoyed this book, would you be kind enough to leave a review for this book on Amazon?

Click here to leave a review for this book on Amazon!

Thank you and good luck!

FIND OUT MORE

Books

DeMolay, Jack. *The Bermuda Triangle: The Disappearance of Flight 19* (Jr. Graphic Mysteries). New York: PowerKids, 2007.

Walker, Kathryn. *The Mystery of Atlantis (Unsolved!)*. New York: Crabtree, 2010.

West, David, and Mike Lacey. *The Bermuda Triangle: Strange Happenings at Sea* (Graphic Mysteries). New York: Rosen, 2006.

Web Sites

adventure.howstuffworks.com/bermuda-triangle.htm
This site explores possible explanations for the Triangle mystery.

www.bermuda-triangle.org/html/introduction_to_the_bermuda_tr.html
This large site was created by a "believer" in the mystery of the Triangle, and it contains many stories of strange events.

www.crystalinks.com/crystalpyr.html
This site was created by a "believer" in the city of Atlantis and its connection to the Triangle mystery.

news.nationalgeographic.com/news/2002/12/1205_021205_bermudatriangle.html
This National Geographic site examines the Bermuda Triangle, discussing key mysterious events and possible explanations.

Movies

Close Encounters of the Third Kind (Columbia: 1977, 2002)
This science fiction movie by Stephen Spielberg is based on the fate of Flight 19.

INDEX